# One Arm Pull Up

Bodyweight Training And
Exercise Program For One Arm
Pull Ups And Chin Ups

Patrick Barrett

Copyright © 2012 Patrick Barrett

All rights reserved.

ISBN-10: 1470108232
ISBN-13: 978-1470108236

# CONTENTS

| | |
|---|---|
| Introduction | 1 |
| You Can Really Hurt Yourself | 5 |
| Pull Up Versus Chin Up | 7 |
| Breathing | 9 |
| Joints | 11 |
| Getting There | 14 |
| Warming Up | 20 |
| Two-Armed Exercises | 26 |
|     Pull Ups | 27 |
|     Slow Pull Ups | 29 |
|     Stutter Pull Ups | 31 |
|     Side-To-Side Pull Ups | 33 |
|     Skinning The Cat | 35 |
|     Midway Hang | 39 |
|     Third-Range Pull Ups | 41 |
|     Biased Midway Hang | 44 |
|     Biased Third-Range Pull Ups | 46 |
|     Biased Pull Ups | 49 |

| | |
|---|---|
| One Arm Exercises | 53 |
|    One Arm Hang | 55 |
|    Assisted One Arm Pull Up | 56 |
|    One Arm Pull Up Negative | 59 |
|    One Arm Midway Hang | 63 |
|    Jumping One Arm Pull Up | 65 |
|    One Arm Pull Up | 68 |
| Reps, Sets, Schedules | 70 |
| Actually Doing A One Arm Pull Up | 75 |
| Nutrition | 77 |
| Conclusion | 80 |
| Books By Patrick Barrett | 82 |
| About The Author | 83 |

"The difference between a successful person and others is not a lack of strength, not a lack of knowledge, but rather a lack of will."

*-Vince Lombardi, iconic world champion NFL coach and Hall of Famer*

**Books by Patrick Barrett:**

*Natural Exercise: Basic Bodyweight Training and Calisthenics for Strength and Weight-Loss*

*The Natural Diet: Simple Nutritional Advice For Optimal Health In The Modern World*

*One Arm Pull Up: Bodyweight Training And Exercise Program For One Arm Pull Ups And Chin Ups*

Disclaimer:

This book was not written or reviewed by a doctor, personal trainer, dietitian, or other licensed person. Always consult with your doctor before beginning any exercise routine or implementing any change in your diet or medication.

# INTRODUCTION

Hi, my name is Patrick Barrett, and I'd like to thank you for buying this book.

The one arm pull up is, quite simply, a very impressive feat—not just of strength, but of overall joint and muscle conditioning, body awareness, and sheer willpower. There are stories of the rare few who are able to perform this skill early and often, usually due to small overall size and early involvement in bodyweight and/or gymnastic training, but for most people the road to the one arm chin up or pull up is long and winding. It's hard, and it takes time.

One of the most difficult aspects of training for the one arm pull up is that, since few people are able to do it, there does not seem to be any kind of established routine for 'getting there.' Most of what you will find online amounts to articles or forum discussions featuring people who can not actually perform the feat themselves, but who list a set of exercises which they 'imagine' will develop the strength you need to do the exercise. When I have seen these articles and discussions, they have been almost universally wrong.

There are, to be fair, a couple of helpful tutorials on the subject online, but I've found them to be insufficient as far as providing a complete picture of what you will need to do to accomplish this feat in a timely manner—and, most importantly, without injury.

I was able to develop the ability to do a one arm pull up through trial and error, on my own, after a longer period of time than was really necessary. I've learned a few things along the way, and I know that if I had access to this resource from the beginning, it would have been a great help to me. I'm glad that I can offer it to you, and I hope you are able to use it to maximum effect.

The one arm pull up is really an exciting exercise, and training for it has value beyond the strength it can provide you—in this process you will learn quite a bit about your muscles, your joints, and your will and dedication to accomplish something difficult.

Nowadays, people often value muscle size and appearance over real strength and health, and the one arm pull up is the exact opposite of that. It's an old-school, hardcore strength exercise, and I hope that together we can help it make a comeback.

Now let's get started.

Books by Patrick Barrett:

*Natural Exercise: Basic Bodyweight Training and Calisthenics for Strength and Weight-Loss*

*The Natural Diet: Simple Nutritional Advice For Optimal Health In The Modern World*

# YOU CAN REALLY HURT YOURSELF

Okay, enough of the motivational stuff. Let's take a minute to evaluate the reality of this situation.

When you train for the one arm pull up, you can really, really hurt yourself. I have to say this for legal reasons, but I also have to say it because it's true. If you do everything right, if you take it slow, if you're smart about it—well, you can still hurt yourself. But you'll be less likely to.

I don't necessarily want to dissuade you from doing this. It can be really gratifying, and I'm certainly glad I spent so much time and effort on it. But it's just a fact, and if you decide you want to give it a shot, you have to realize that and take responsibility for it. This kind of training can result in injury.

One of the biggest reasons that you might hurt yourself, and one of the biggest challenges to overcome in training for this exercise, is instability. With two hands on the pull up bar, you not only have the strength of both arms, you have the stability of two points of contact.

In a one arm pull up or chin up, you're only touching the bar in one place, which creates the potential for swinging and twisting during the movement. When you add swinging and twisting into the equation along with extreme muscular strain, you've got a recipe for some ugly injuries.

Incidentally, this stability issue is one of the reasons that training for a one arm pull up or chin up is not as simple as training to do a regular pull up with the equivalent of your bodyweight hanging from a weight belt around your waist. In other words, some people think that a person who weighs 150 pounds and trains to do a regular pull up while loaded down with 150 pounds of extra weight should be able to do a one arm pull up as well, because they assume being able to do a two-armed pull up with 300 pounds means you can do a one arm pull up with 150 pounds.

That's a great goal to have, and an impressive thing to do, but it's only a piece of the puzzle, and that alone will not get you there.

A person who can do a pull up at double bodyweight is certainly closer to the one arm pull up than someone who can't even come close, but I personally don't recommend weighted pull ups as training to people who are trying to do one arm pull ups—not because they can't make you a lot stronger or because they're bad, but simply because they aren't the most direct way to go about it. For that reason, it's not something we'll discuss further in this book.

Furthermore, I'd prefer to teach you how to achieve this goal without any special props or equipment other than a pull up bar, so you won't need to buy a weight belt, or plates, or elastic bands, or anything like that.

You can approach this intelligently, and you can greatly minimize all of these risks, but there will always be a risk of injury there. There is, of course, some risk of injury whenever you do any kind of training, or anything else for that matter; risk is a part of life.

However, the risks of training for a one arm pull up, particularly when you're doing the exercises that only involve one hand on the pull up bar, are not insignificant.

Like I said, this doesn't necessarily mean you should give up. However, it does mean that you need to take this seriously. I will do everything I can to teach you a reasonable progression so that you aren't rushing into anything you can't handle, but there will necessarily be points in the training where you will have to take that 'leap' into something new, and a little more difficult, and risky.

You must take this risk seriously, and you must be sure not to move ahead too quickly into something you can't handle. Always take baby steps, and never cut corners. You'll learn the details you'll need to be able to do that in the coming chapters, but for now just keep it in mind.

Be patient, and be smart. It's worth it.

## PULL UP VERSUS CHIN UP

Throughout this book I will talk for the most part about the 'one arm pull up,' but there is, of course, also the one arm chin up.

For the pull up, the palm of the hand gripping the bar will face away from your armpit. For the chin up, the palm of the hand gripping the bar will face toward your armpit.

The difference is not extremely important; one is not really harder or easier than the other across the board. Some people will feel naturally inclined to do one over the other, and if you find yourself to be more comfortable with one of them, then that's fine—there's certainly no reason to make this any harder on yourself than it already is. Once you make it with the first one, it will just take a little bit more training to get the other one.

However, I would recommend even if you tend to work with one grip, still do some work with the other grip. Working both ways will lay a good foundation and will help you to overcome the stability issues we talked about earlier, and will talk about again later in the book.

The differences in the training are, for the most part, obvious, and on the rare occasion that there is an important reason to differentiate the two, I will do that.

For now, though, you don't need to worry. Once you start working with one arm, you'll probably find one grip feels more 'natural' than the other. You should work with both, although it's okay to tend more toward one than the other. Once you get there with one grip, just expand your training to include more of the other variation.

## BREATHING

Breathing is an extremely important and often overlooked aspect of any exercise, and if you want to progress on the one arm pull up then you will need to be very aware of your breathing.

As is almost always the case, you will be exhaling on the more difficult part of the movement.

On exercises that focus on a pull up motion, that will be the pull up.

On exercises that focus on a negative, you will exhale slowly during the negative.

On exercises that focus on holding one position, you will exhale slowly while you try to hold that position as long as possible.

The one arm pull up is, for most people, an all-out type of exercise—it's not something you're probably going to do twenty of, and obviously in the beginning your goal is just to work your way up to one.

A lot of the exercises you do leading up to it will also push your limits as you do just one, or two, or three reps. Each rep is intense, and each rep requires you to focus—and each rep also requires you to breathe correctly.

Before you attempt any exercise, for the first time or otherwise, one of the things you need to get straight is your breathing. Ready yourself so that when you need your strength most, you will be able to exhale strongly during the exertion.

If this sounds strange now, don't worry. Keep it in mind as you begin the exercises and it will become second nature.

## JOINTS

Taking care of your joints is critical in any exercise, but it is perhaps most critical when you pursue the one arm pull up.

I've said it before, I'll say it again: you can really mess up your joints with this exercise. You're going to be subjecting your wrist, elbow, and shoulder to forces they have not seen before, and it will not always be comfortable or, to be honest, pain-free.

Knowing the proper way to handle this situation is critical.

Most people who exercise regularly understand the process by which muscle is developed. When you engage in intense exercise, your muscles work hard and end up breaking down a little bit. Once you're done, your body recovers, and repairs the broken-down muscle. After it repairs the muscle, it becomes a little bit stronger.

If you repeat this process over and over again, you can increase your muscular strength significantly.

Like I said, most people know that. However, did you know that the same process can work on your joints?

Joints, just like muscles, can be strengthened and developed. They can be trained to perform better in the future than they do now.

So if you try some of these more difficult exercises and experience discomfort—even discomfort bordering on pain—that doesn't mean you won't be able to do them, it just means you have to be careful and condition your joints, just like you condition your muscles, so that they will be able to handle the extra load.

I've heard from some people who say that trying to do a one arm pull up is stupid, that it's an unnatural exercise, and that the joints in your arm just can't handle the forces involved. This is unreasonable on its surface, simply because there are many people who have been able to perform the exercise, and their joints are clearly handling the forces involved.

The other reason that it makes no sense is that it discounts your body's ability to adapt your joints to new situations. Of course a person who hasn't done any one arm pull up training will have joints that are unready for that kind of exercise. But once that person trains correctly and intelligently, his joints will become ready.

It's as simple as that.

The key difference between conditioning muscles and conditioning joints is time. Muscles can recover in a matter of days, but joints can take weeks or months to adapt to new levels of stress in new situations.

That means that if you're serious about attaining this skill, you need to be patient. That's so important that I'll make it its own paragraph.

Be patient.

In most situations your workout ends when you are no longer able to perform an exercise because your muscles aren't able to continue. However, when training for the one arm pull up—especially in the first few weeks or months—you will often end a workout because your joints are unable to continue.

You might feel, from a purely muscular standpoint, that you could try for another rep or two. However, if you start to feel discomfort or too much strain on your wrist, elbow, shoulder, wherever—that's when you need to call it a day.

It can be frustrating because you might feel like you could force out a few more reps and just 'deal' with the pain in your joints, but if you do that, you're asking for trouble. Your joints will come along, and they will get conditioned to the point that it's not really an issue anymore.

But in the beginning, you need to be smart and cut short your one arm pull up workout if your joints start to feel strained or uncomfortable.

Be patient.

# GETTING THERE

Training for a one arm pull up or one arm chin up is a process. There are a lot of variables and a lot of 'little things' to be aware of, which I will try to cover in this chapter.

First of all, this kind of training will not be the same for everyone. As a general rule, the taller you are and the heavier you are, the more difficult this will be—taller people will tend to have longer arms and a longer distance to move their bodies, and heavier people will obviously be moving more weight.

However, no matter how tall or heavy you are, there is almost certainly someone taller and heavier than you who has done a one arm pull up before you, so don't be discouraged.

If you are on the taller or heavier side, you will still take all the same steps to get there; they will probably just take more time. I'm about 5'11" and 195 pounds—not the tallest or heaviest guy in the world, but on the bigger side of most people doing one arm pull ups.

If you're 5'5" and 130 pounds, then you're obviously in a better position to get there faster, and you probably will spend less time having to wait for your joint conditioning to catch up with your muscular conditioning, and that sort of thing.

However, it's very important that you remember that you're not going to change how tall you are or where you're starting from. Whether you feel you have a size advantage or a size disadvantage, the answer if you want to progress is still the same—train as hard and smart as you can, and be patient and disciplined.

One thing to keep in mind, though, is your weight. If you weigh 200 pounds because you're in good shape and that's just how much you weigh, then that's fine and it's nothing to worry about. However, if you weigh 200 pounds because you're thirty pounds overweight, then that's obviously going to make things more difficult for you.

Every pound you lose is a pound you don't have to lift with one arm. That doesn't mean it's worth it, or at all advisable, to develop some kind of eating disorder and try to shed every pound possible, but if you're carrying around a lot of extra weight, you obviously need to work on that as much as you work on getting stronger.

Don't take it the wrong way—if you're not carrying around much extra weight, then don't starve yourself to drop weight, and don't spend any time worrying about this. A few pounds is not that important, and the energy you lose starving yourself will leave you worse off anyway.

But if you're 20 pounds overweight and you're serious about being able to do a one arm pull up or chin up, losing that weight is as important as your pull up training.

There will be times when you feel like you're not making any progress. That's fine. Every time you have a good work out and don't injure yourself, you've taken a step forward, whether it feels like it or not.

Depending on your physical size and current condition, your diet, and your schedule, this process could take several months. There will be a lot of times when you're just grinding away. Stick with it.

The one arm pull up is not just a pull up that is twice as hard. It is its own skill. Obviously the two are related, and obviously there's some overlap in the training and technique, but you need to realize that you're also learning something new.

Because you only have one point of contact with the bar, you will have to learn to find stability at every point in the movement. Your body will twist slightly in toward your hand as you go up, and it will twist slightly outward away from your hand as you go down.

You will learn to stick your free arm forward and slightly out from your body for balance, and you will also learn how to hold your legs on the way up and down.

Little things like this are why I prefer to do a lot of training focusing on one arm on a real pull up bar (as opposed to a two arm exercise, or using a device that offers assistance).

Some people might want to use an assisted pullup machine with one arm, and just use less assistance over time until they don't need any help. If you try this, you'll most likely find that you make a little 'progress' in the very beginning, and then soon hit a point that you absolutely can not get past.

That's because the assisted pull up machine takes you through a motion that has very little in common with an actual one arm pull up.

Others will recommend that you use resistance bands, levers, ropes, or towels to assist you in different ways as you try to approach the one arm pull up. These techniques are better than using the assisted pull up machine, and they will actually allow you to progress toward your goal. If you are very conscientious as you do them, and you know just the right motion to go through, they can definitely be beneficial.

However, they are not the approach that I recommend, because they still change the path that your body goes through as you attempt the exercise, which can lead to picking up bad habits, and, just as importantly, not picking up the good habits you would develop if you were working with one arm only.

I've seen articles online mention that if you're going to do a one arm pull up, you should attempt it right in the beginning of your workout, because it will be the most difficult thing you do, so you want to be as fresh as possible.

This is inaccurate. Because of the tremendous strain involved—particularly if you are of average size or larger—you need to be a lot 'warmer' than you might need to be for another exercise.

For example, I've actually found that a one arm pull up can be easier after an hour of climbing at the rock gym, simply because all of the muscles in your arm, shoulder, and back are so completely warmed up that they are more ready to do the motion.

You may find out that your attempts at the one arm pull up are more successful after not just a regular warm up, but also a set, or two, or three, of regular pull ups.

We'll talk about the specifics when we talk about the exercises, and (more importantly) you'll also be able to get a good idea from seeing the way I do it in the pictures. The most important thing, though, is that you'll pick up on these things as you try it yourself.

You need to realize, though, that when you start doing some of these basic exercises for the first time, you might feel more lost than you expect. You might do something and feel like you were totally out of control, and here's why: you're trying do something that seems simple, but actually involves a number of different smaller skills that you're going to have to nail down.

In the beginning, your joints won't be ready, you won't be able to control yourself, up or down, to keep from twisting the wrong way, you won't know the way you actually should be twisting, you won't know where to put your other arm, or your legs. It will all be new to you, and it will all come with a little practice.

Just continue using the progression I show you, continue being patient and disciplined, and—this is very important if you want to make progress—pay attention to your body while you do the exercises. Think about which way it's trying to lean or twist, and correct for it. You need to

## One Arm Pull Up

develop that awareness every bit as much as you need to develop muscular strength.

You know what was the sorest part of me after I did my first one arm chin up negative? My abs. By far. Next was my bicep. That's not what I expected, but it's what happened. Don't go into this assuming you know how it's going to be.

Pay as much attention to as many of the details as you can. It will make you feel lost for a little while in the beginning, but if you keep working at it, things will start to come together.

# WARMING UP

As I briefly mentioned in the previous chapter, warming up properly is a critical component of your one arm pull up workout for two reasons:

1. It will help you to perform the best you can by preparing all of the necessary muscle groups for the strain they will endure.

2. It will help to keep you from injuring yourself during the workout.

Now, I know those things are true of warming up for any exercise, but they are especially true when you start training for the one arm pull up. You will need to make sure that you are thoroughly warm whenever you do train for this skill, and that means not just the normal set of light exercises, but also a few sets of actual pull ups.

## One Arm Pull Up

In general, the larger you are and the more strain you're putting on your joints and muscles, the longer the warm up needs to be.

Before a one arm pull up workout, you should do any combination of stretching and warming up that you would regularly do. Personally, I like a warm up that includes a few sets of toe touches and jumping jacks.

Then add these two movements to further warm up your arms and shoulder joints:

1. Stand with your arms extended up. Keeping your arms extended through the entire movement, swing them out in front of you, and then down by your sides, then continue to keep them extended as you let the momentum carry your arms behind you. Then bring them down, then forward, then straight up again.

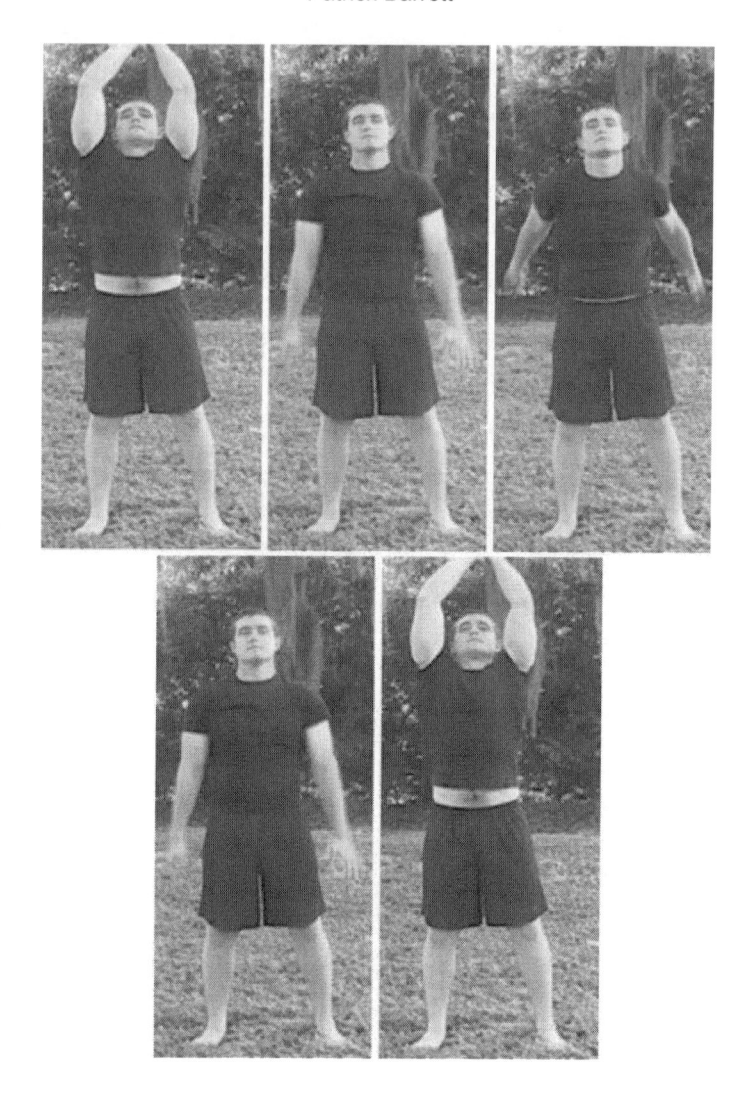

Continue this in one smooth, controlled motion, swinging your arms up, then forward, down, and back, then down, forward and up, back and forth, for one or two sets of 10-

## One Arm Pull Up

20 reps. This will help to loosen and warm up your shoulder joints.

2. Stand with your arms straight out to either side, like a 'T.' Keeping your arms straight, bring them in across your chest. Then swing them back out again, until you are back in the T position, and let their momentum carry your arms even a little behind your body.

Keeping your arms straight, swing your arms forward across your chest again, and repeat. Note in the pictures how I alternate which arm is on top when my arms cross, for the sake of keeping things even.

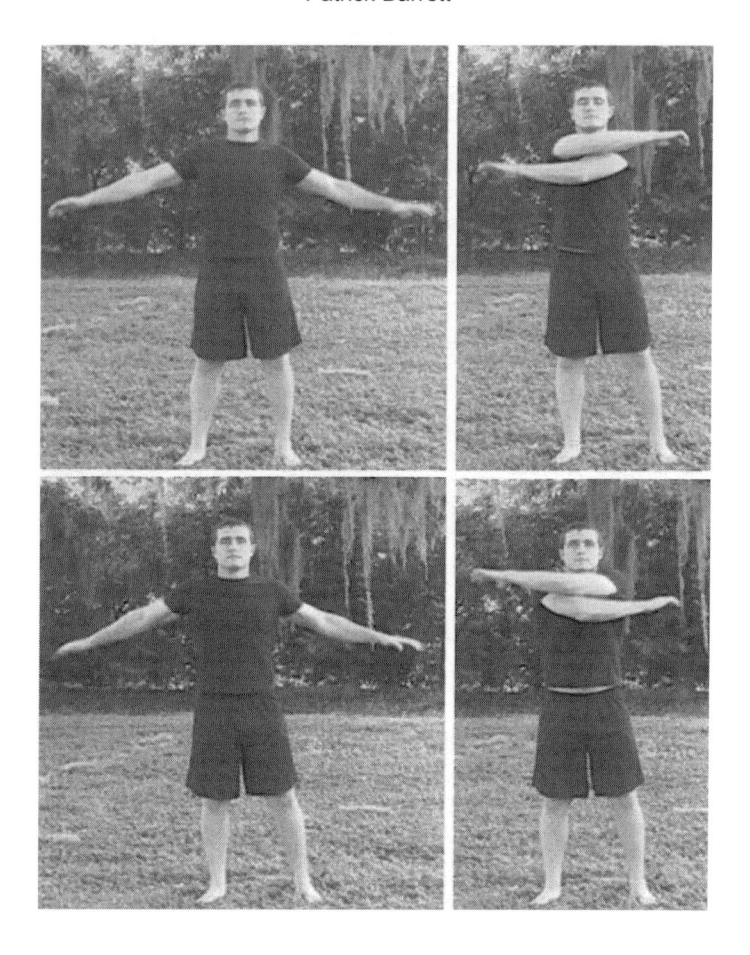

You should do this in one smooth, fluid, controlled motion, swinging your arms across your chest, then straight out to the sides and back, then back forward again. Repeat this movement for one or two sets of 10-20 reps. This will help to warm up and loosen your arms and your shoulder joints.

After that, you'll want to perform anywhere from one to three sets of 5-12 pull ups or chin ups. You may even want

## One Arm Pull Up

to throw in a couple of slower pull ups within those sets, and maybe hold the up position for a few seconds during the sets too.

Just go through that pull up motion quite a few times, and don't rush it—feel your muscles doing the work, and getting the warmth and blood flow that you're going to need when you start trying to work with one arm.

Once you're much more used to all this, and especially once your joints adapt to the strain, you won't need quite as long a warmup before the workout, but even now I always do a good warm up and the arm swinging exercises, and at least one set of 8-12 pull ups (with a slow rep or two in there) before I get into the various one arm exercises.

A good warm up is critical. Don't overlook it.

## TWO-ARMED EXERCISES

You want to spend a lot of your time training for the one arm pull up by doing exercises that use, or at least focus on, just one arm. However, before you get there, you need to prepare yourself by training with a variety of two arm pull up exercises that are designed to build up strength in your whole upper body.

The exercises toward the end of this list can also be quite effective at training for the one arm pull up or chin up—even though they use two arms—as long as you are careful about your form.

## PULL UPS

You probably have these figured out by now. Be sure to pull all the way up until your chin is well clear of the bar, and be sure to go all the way down until your arms are extended. Don't cheat yourself on the range of motion, because you'll need the whole range to do the one arm variety.

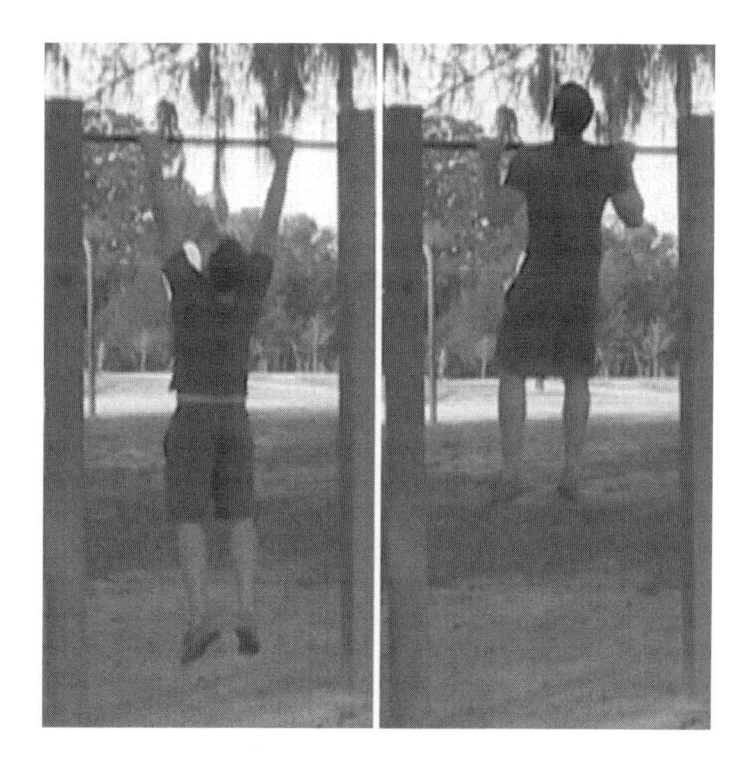

## SLOW PULL UPS

Slower pull ups will build strength along the entire normal range of the pull up motion.

As you might imagine, slow pull ups are just like ordinary pull ups, except you slow down the movement considerably.

Don't cheat. Stay slow from the bottom all the way to the top, and from the top back down to the bottom. If you don't work to keep the same speed all the way through, you won't build even strength all the way through, so keep yourself honest.

Deciding your number of reps can be a little difficult here, because it depends on exactly how slow you're going. Obviously, doing one pull up that takes two minutes is going to be harder than three pull ups that you do in one minute total.

You can do a set of a few slow pull ups, you can do just one very, very slow pull up, or you can add in a slow pull up during or at the end of a set of normal pull ups.

These are also a good idea in the warming up phase of your workout because slowing down makes sure you hit every little muscle group in the whole range of motion.

## STUTTER PULL UPS

The stutter pull up has the same range of motion as a normal pull up. However, the difference is that during the range of motion, you stop, completely, several times.

The idea is that the pull up gets a lot harder, and the workout gets a lot better, when you've got way less momentum on your side. Stopping completely over and over again (just for an instant) strengthens you throughout the whole movement.

You can stop four or five times, or you can stop 20 times or more. When I do this exercise I usually 'stutter' maybe 10 or 15 times. To be honest, I don't count them, I just stop every inch or two on my way up, and every inch or two on my way down. I almost always stutter on the way up and down, but to change it up sometimes you can do them only on the way up, or only on the way down.

As with the slow pull ups, you are the one who determines how hard each rep is, and one rep can be much more challenging than three or four depending on how difficult you make them. The same idea applies—you can do one, or a few, or mix them in to a set of normal pull ups, or a warm up (or all of the above).

## SIDE-TO-SIDE PULL UPS

This is the first exercise where you'll start working each arm separately. Just assume a slightly wider pull up (or chin up) grip, and then pull yourself up toward one hand, then down again, then up toward the other hand, then down again. Always remember to work both sides evenly.

As you can see in the pictures, your weight at the bottom of the pull up is distributed evenly from left to right, and you only start to pull in one direction or the other as you pull yourself up.

Patrick Barrett

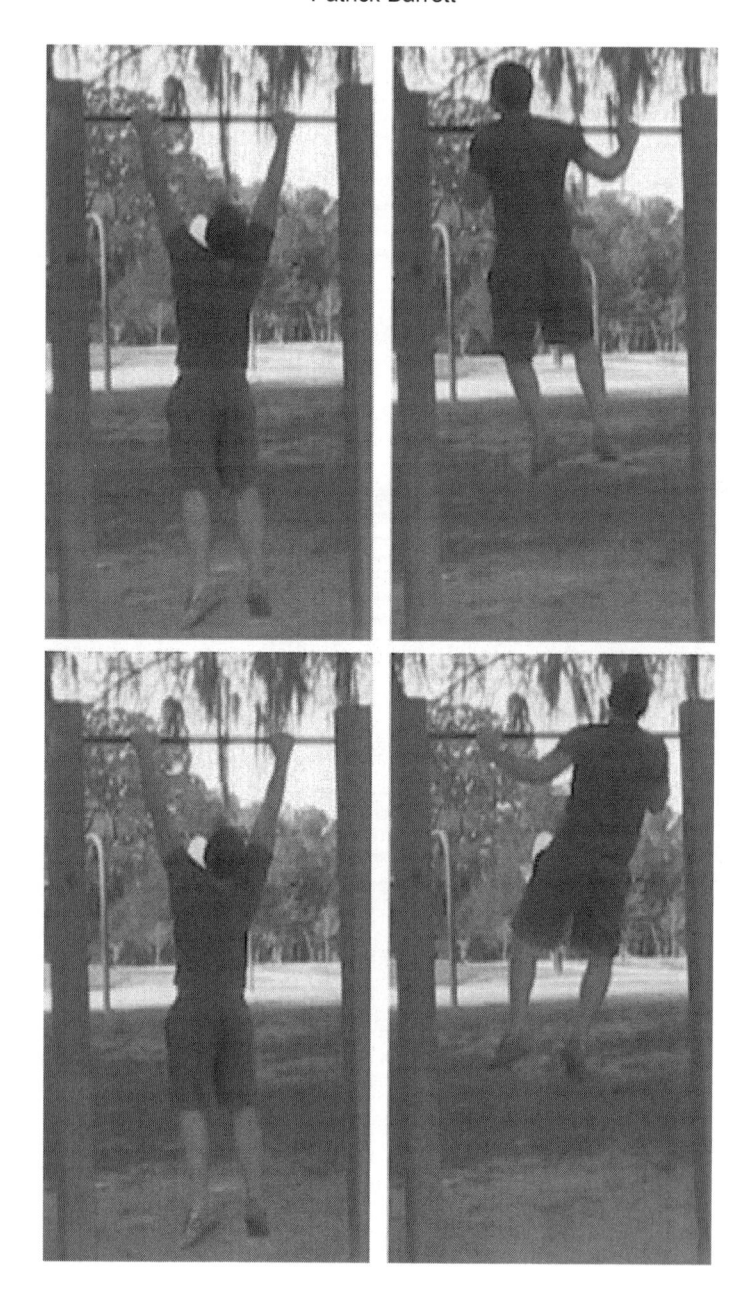

## SKINNING THE CAT

This is one of the stranger exercises, and it's going to make some people a little nervous. It's not absolutely necessary, so if you aren't comfortable with it, then feel free to skip it. However, if you think you'd like to give it a shot, it's one that I like a lot, and it can really stretch and open up and activate some muscles in your shoulder and armpit area that are hard to hit otherwise.

You're going to start hanging from the bar. Next, bring your knees up into your chest. Then, start to lean back and bring your lower body up toward the bar. You may need to cross your feet to allow them to fit under the bar as your bring your legs through your arms.

Once you've brought your legs through your arms, you may slowly lower your legs to maximize the stretch in your shoulders, as shown in the fifth image.

Let me make it clear that this exercise is done slowly and methodically. You don't swing your legs up and through your arms and flip over all of a sudden; the whole thing should be done slowly and in complete control, in every part of the motion from start to finish.

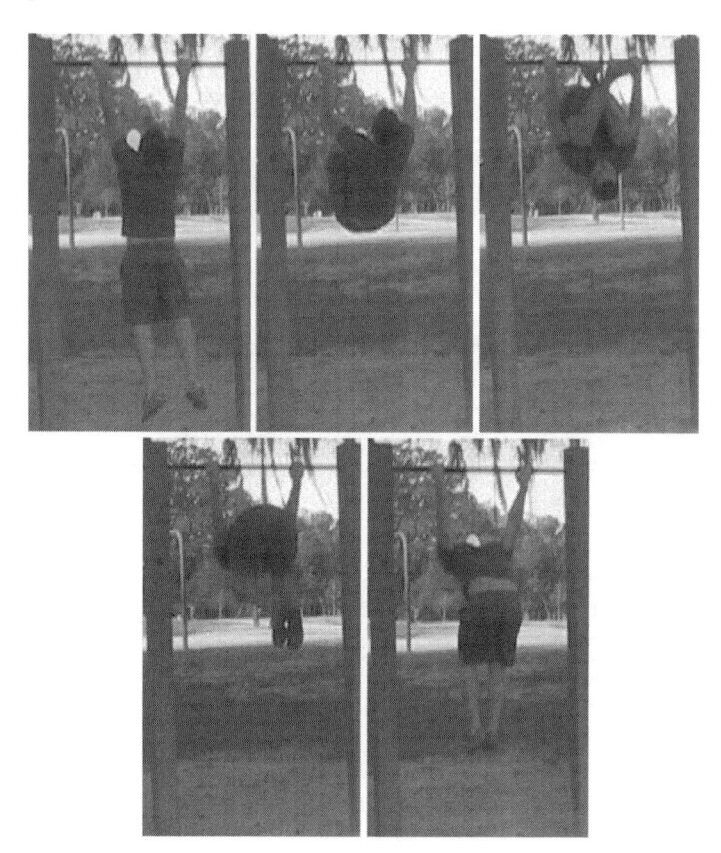

To do this exercise, you have to be comfortable with the positions you'll be putting yourself in. As always, adjusting to this new exercise means progressing incrementally. Start by just bringing your knees up into your chest—make sure you're strong enough to do that with control.

## One Arm Pull Up

Then, bring your legs up and start to bring them through your arms, maybe halfway between the second and third pictures, with your back more or less parallel to the ground. Stop before your feet clear the bar, and lower yourself back down.

Become comfortable and confident with this motion. Once you feel good about going this far, you can start to bring your legs through your arm and progress more and more through the motion.

Eventually you should be able to end up in the position shown in the fifth picture. If you've followed the progression as described above, you should not have a problem reversing the same motion you followed to get there, and ending up back in the position in the first picture in the series (hanging from the bar in the usual manner).

However, you can also dismount by simply letting go of the bar with both hands AT THE SAME TIME and just landing on your feet.

Once you've made it all the way through to the position shown in the fifth picture, you can either hold that position as a stretch, and then return to the starting point and get off the bar, or, if you're more adventurous, you can come all the way through, then go back to the starting position, and then come all the way through again, and repeat for several repetitions.

Do not attempt to do multiple repetitions if you aren't already quite comfortable doing one full repetition.

If you ever feel like you're going to fall off, remember two things: let go of both hands (not just one) and try not to land on your head or neck.

Let me point out again here that this exercise is helpful but by no means necessary. Some people will take to this quite naturally, and some people will feel uncomfortable from the start. If you don't feel comfortable trying this, don't spend any time worrying about it, just move on to the next exercise.

Be careful if you try this one.

## MIDWAY HANG

I think hangs are a great way to build up strength at some of the more critical points in the pull up motion. We're going to look at hangs at three main areas:

**Bottom Hang**
Hold this position at the very bottom of the pull up motion when there is still tension through your back and arm. Do not relax all the way to a normal hang where just your forearms are engaged. Your arm should be slightly bent, and your forearm, biceps, and back should all be engaged.

**Middle Hang**
Hold this position with your upper arm parallel to the ground.

**Top Hang**
Hold this position with your chin as high above the bar as possible.

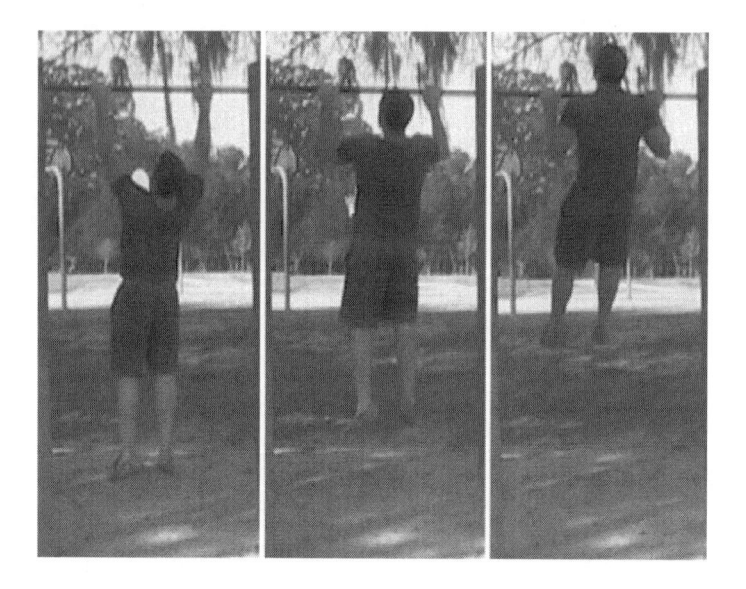

In each case, you're going to hold the position until you start to drop from it involuntarily. Then lower all the way to the bottom, and (optional) do a full pull up, all the way up and down, and then get off the bar.

Unless you notice a major deficiency at one point in particular, always be sure to work all three positions evenly—for each time you do one hang, do the other two as well.

# THIRD-RANGE PULL UPS

This is another way to focus your efforts on the different parts of the pull up motion and build better overall pull up strength.

### Bottom Third Pull Up
You'll do mini pull ups through the bottom third of the movement, from when your arms are just engaged (as in the Bottom Hang) to just below when your upper arm is parallel to the ground.

### Middle Third Pull Up
You'll do mini pull ups through the middle third of the movement, from just below when your upper arm is parallel to the ground to just above when your upper arm is parallel to the ground.

### Top Third Pull Up
You'll do mini pull ups through the top third of the range of motion, from just above when your upper arm is parallel to the ground, to the very top of the movement.

Patrick Barrett

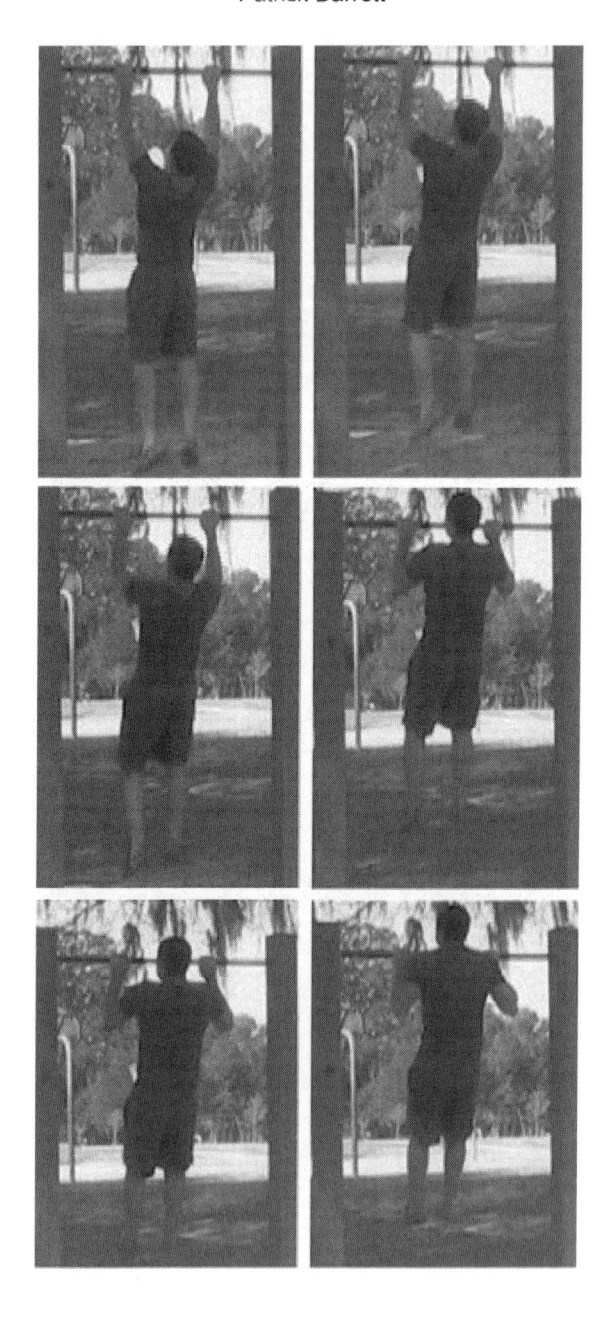

## One Arm Pull Up

Take a look at the pictures—the top row shows the "down" and "up" positions for the bottom third pull up, the middle row shows the "down" and "up" positions for the middle third pull up, and the bottom row shows the "down" and "up" positions for the top third pull up.

For this exercise, I recommend stringing them all together, and I usually do a full pull up in between. Here's an example:

Hang from the bar. Do one pull up all the way up. On the way down, stop in the Bottom Third Pull Up position and do four Bottom Third Pull Ups. Then, do another full pull up, and on the way down stop at the bottom position of the Middle Third Pull Up. Do four of these pull ups, then go all the way down and do another full pull up. From the top position of that pull up, do four of the Top Third Pull Ups, then lower yourself all the way and do one final full pull up, all the way up and down.

Realize that you're staying on the bar that entire time, so it's like doing one 'exercise' with three components. You're basically doing four repetitions of each of the three variations, with a full pull up before and after, and between each variation.

The order you do them in is not that important, though it's probably a good idea to change it up just for the sake of variety. Just be sure to work out each variation evenly. In this example I used four reps at each position, but of course that number will vary; whatever that number is, though, do the same number at the top, middle, and bottom.

## BIASED MIDWAY HANG

This is just like the Midway Hang, with a subtle and important difference. You're going to shift your weight so that you're holding as much as possible with one arm and not the other. That's going to train your arms independently to work hard and get stronger.

The three positions are the same. For each one, get into the normal hang. Then, shift your weight to the side you're working first. Hold that until you can feel that your arm is no longer able to hold most of the weight. Then, shift straight over to the other arm and hold that one for as long as you can.

You will probably only be able to do each one for a few seconds. If you can do more than a few seconds, then shift more of your weight over to that arm. Afterward, (optional) drop all the way to the bottom and do a full pull up, up and down.

## One Arm Pull Up

After you've done the hang from one position on both arms, drop of the bar, rest for a minute or so, then get back on the bar and do the next position on both arms, then drop off and rest again, and then get back on and do the final position on each arm.

Always be sure to work both arms evenly, and be sure to work each position evenly too. Feel free to change up the order in which you do them.

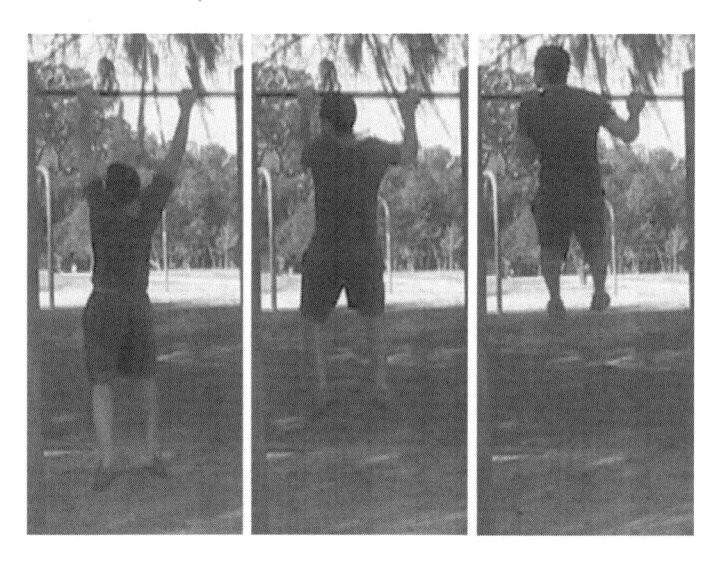

Alternate which arm you start with from workout to workout. In other words, if you work your right arm first and then your left, next time around work your left first, then your right.

## BIASED THIRD-RANGE PULL UPS

As you might expect, these are just like the Third Range Pull Ups we discussed earlier, except you'll be leaning to one side as you do them in order to target that side more directly. Then, once you're done on the first side, you'll immediately shift your weight to the other side to hit that one.

Look at the pictures—the top row shows the biased "down" and "up" positions for the bottom third pull up, the middle row shows the biased "down" and "up" positions for the middle third pull up, and the bottom row shows the biased "down" and "up" positions for the top third pull up.

Just take the normal Third Range Pull Up sequence, and divide each variation into two halves where you shift your weight so most of the burden is on the one side, and then shift so most is on the other.

# One Arm Pull Up

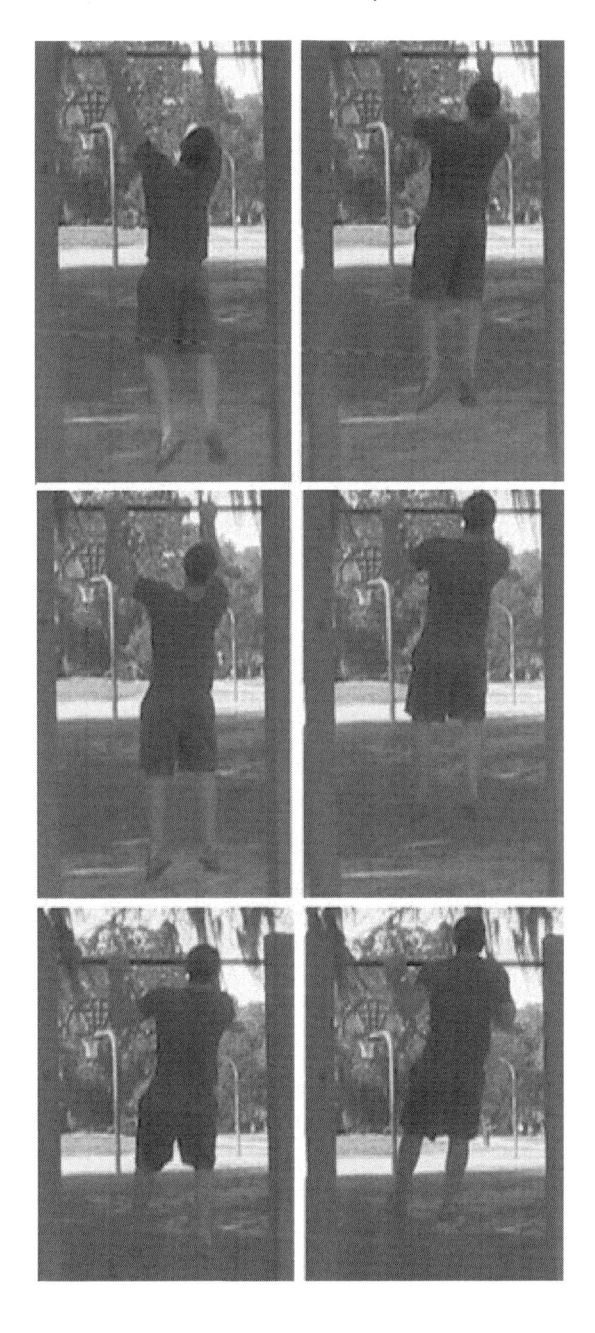

Whether you're at the bottom, middle, or lower part of the range, you'll do the left and right sides right in a row. In other words, don't do the whole sequence on your right side, and then the whole sequence on your left. Instead, do the left side of the lower range, then the right side; the left side of the middle range, then the right side; then the left side of the upper range, then the right.

Feel free to change up the order of left/right and top/middle/bottom, just make sure you work out everything evenly.

## BIASED PULL UPS

If you can be 'honest' with these pull ups, and work as hard as you can to simulate working with one arm, these can be one of the most effective tools you use on your path toward the one arm pull up.

The basic idea is that you complete a full pull up motion focusing on one arm and minimizing your use of the other arm. The two most important elements are (1) accurately simulating (as best you can) the movement of pulling up with one arm, and (2) effectively minimizing the help you get from the other arm.

Obviously you need some help from that arm, because you can't do a pull up yet without it, but you need to make sure that you're getting the minimum amount of help you can stand while still executing the pull up.

As far as the first element goes, the best way to make sure that you're following the right 'path' is to look carefully at the pictures, and also to notice the way your body travels on the one arm pull up negatives (you'll get to those soon).

Basically, you want to start the motion with your chin up against the shoulder of the main arm, and more or less below the main hand, and you want to move your chin in a straight line up to—or perhaps right next to—that hand.

For the second part of the equation, you need to pay attention. You can feel if you're using one arm much more than the other or not. The next thing is to follow the right path, as described above, because to some extent that will force you to use that arm more.

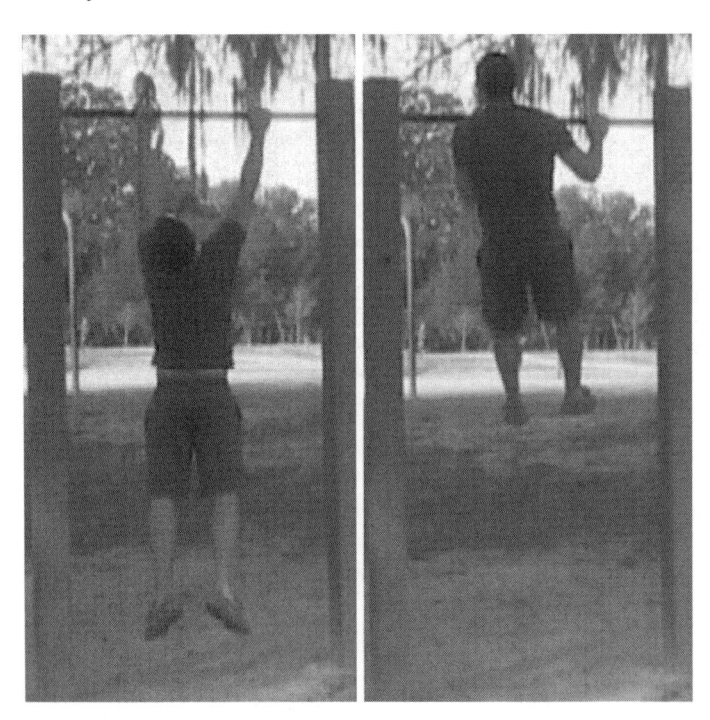

## One Arm Pull Up

Another thing you can do is experiment with different hand positions for your secondary hand that will force it to contribute less to the movement. One way to do this is use fewer fingers. If you've only got two fingers, or one finger, on the bar, most people are not going to be able to get much strength out of that hand.

Don't go crazy and push it by using just a pinky or anything, because you don't want to pull or tear anything in your hand, but try using your index and middle fingers, or your middle and ring fingers. If you think you're up to it, try with just your index finger, or just your middle finger; just be cautious.

The other thing you can do is move your secondary hand farther away down the bar. This can be very effective, but only if you keep your weight under the primary hand—otherwise, you're just doing a wider grip pull up with both arms. Stay under your main hand, and the bad angle on your other arm will force you to use your main arm to lift yourself.

As you progress, you can also combine the two—move your secondary arm farther away, and also only use one or two fingers on that hand.

However, it's not really necessary to move your arm away or use fewer fingers if you can make sure you're honest with yourself about using your main arm to lift yourself as much as possible. If you prefer using all the fingers on your secondary hand, and not moving it too far away, that can be fine, given that you're still using as much of your primary arm as possible.

For this exercise, you should work one arm at a time—in other words, once you do a whole set focusing on one arm, you should drop off the bar, give yourself a minute or so to recover, and then get back up and do the other arm. Also, whether you're using the pull up or chin up grip on your primary hand, you should use the pull up grip (palm forward) on your secondary hand; in my experience, that just makes it easier to complete the motion correctly.

Remember, this should be tough. If you're able to approach ten reps on this exercise, you're either getting very close to doing the one arm pull up, or you aren't doing them right because you're giving yourself too much help with your other arm. Be strict with yourself.

## ONE ARM EXERCISES

Along with the biased pull ups, these are going to be your primary weapons as you strive toward the one arm pull up or chin up. Since you have only one arm on the bar at a time, they are considerably less stable, which makes them considerably more risky with regard to injury. Be patient and careful.

If it's your first time doing an exercise, give yourself plenty of time to get comfortable with it and to get the form right. Read the instructions and look at the pictures carefully, and don't rush into anything. Depending on your size and physical condition, shifting to one arm can be a considerable change, so take it seriously.

You're obviously going to be working out one arm at a time, since you're only using one arm at a time. For each exercise, do a full set on one arm, get down from the bar, give yourself a minute's rest, and then do your full set on your other arm.

Try to vary which arm you work first from workout to workout—it's not a huge deal, but it's always best to work for balance on both sides of your body, especially when you're only working one side at a time.

For each of these exercises, you're going to continue doing reps until you can't do another rep in control and with good form. That might mean seven reps, and it might mean one rep. Just keep doing it until you can't do it the right way any more (or, of course, until you experience any joint pain, in which case you should call it a day).

Oh, and I always try to do the same number of reps on each arm. You can make an argument either way about this, but if I can do five reps of something on one arm, I do five on the other arm, even if I feel like I could maybe do six on the second arm. You will almost certainly find that one arm is stronger than the other, but I like to work for balance, which means keeping the reps even on both sides as best you can.

# ONE ARM HANG

This is pretty straightforward—if you're going to do a one arm pull up, you're going to need to be able to hang from the bar with one arm in a controlled manner. This isn't going to be the cornerstone of your workout or anything, but it can be good to throw in a hang for as long as you can on each hand near the end of a workout.

You want to hang in a way that matches up with the way you will be at the bottom of a one arm pull up or chin up, you don't just want to hang completely relaxed, and uncontrolled, and twisting from side to side. You'll be able to feel more of what that means as you work with the other one arm exercises.

## ASSISTED ONE ARM PULL UP

The easier form of this exercise is often confused with a one arm pull up or chin up, when in fact it should be called a one hand pull up, since you're still using the strength of both arms.

At any rate, this can be an interesting and useful exercise of varying difficulty. The basic idea is that you help out your main arm with your secondary arm by putting your secondary arm on your main arm, as shown in the picture.

A lot of people have seen this where you grab your main wrist with your secondary hand, but they are not aware that you can change the amount of help you get by changing your hand placement, as shown in the pictures. There are four basic hand placements, which I will list here in order of increasing difficulty:

Hand Placement 1) Grip your primary wrist with your secondary hand.

## One Arm Pull Up

Hand Placement 2) Slide your hand down about six inches from its placement in (1), so that your secondary hand is grabbing the thickest part of your primary forearm.

Hand Placement 3) Place your secondary hand on your primary bicep, and slide it in toward the crook of your elbow.

Hand Placement 4) Place your secondary hand on your primary deltoid, so that the outside edge of your hand is laying where your deltoid ends and your bicep begins.

If you can do a couple of pull ups from hand placement 4, you have made good progress toward doing a one arm pull up.

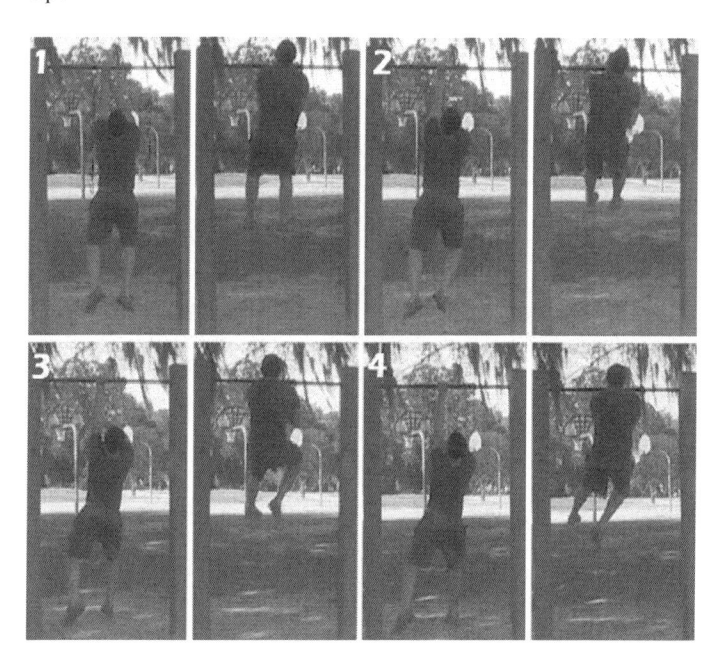

When you first approach this exercise, experiment with your secondary arm at each different point to see where you stand. Once you incorporate it into a workout, start on the most difficult variation you can do at least one full rep of on each arm.

After you can't do another rep of that variation, wait a minute or so and move to the next most difficult, do as many as you can on each arm, then move to the next most difficult.

## ONE ARM PULL UP NEGATIVE

This is a big step in your progression—being able to lower yourself in a controlled manner from the top of a one arm pull up or chin up all the way down to the bottom. Some people swear by these, and they have always been a primary component of my one arm pull up workouts.

These will become second nature, but for the first several workouts you want to pay attention to all the details to make sure you get it right and don't hurt yourself. You're going to pull yourself up with both hands (1), and then pause for a moment at the top of the motion. Shift your weight toward your primary hand. Consciously think about and engage all of the muscles involved—your hand, forearm, bicep, back, abs—feel them holding all of your weight (2). Then, take a deep, steady breath, release your other hand (3), and lower yourself in a slow, controlled manner while you exhale in a slow, controlled manner (4). Once you've lowered yourself all the way, put your secondary hand back on the bar, and then get back on the ground.

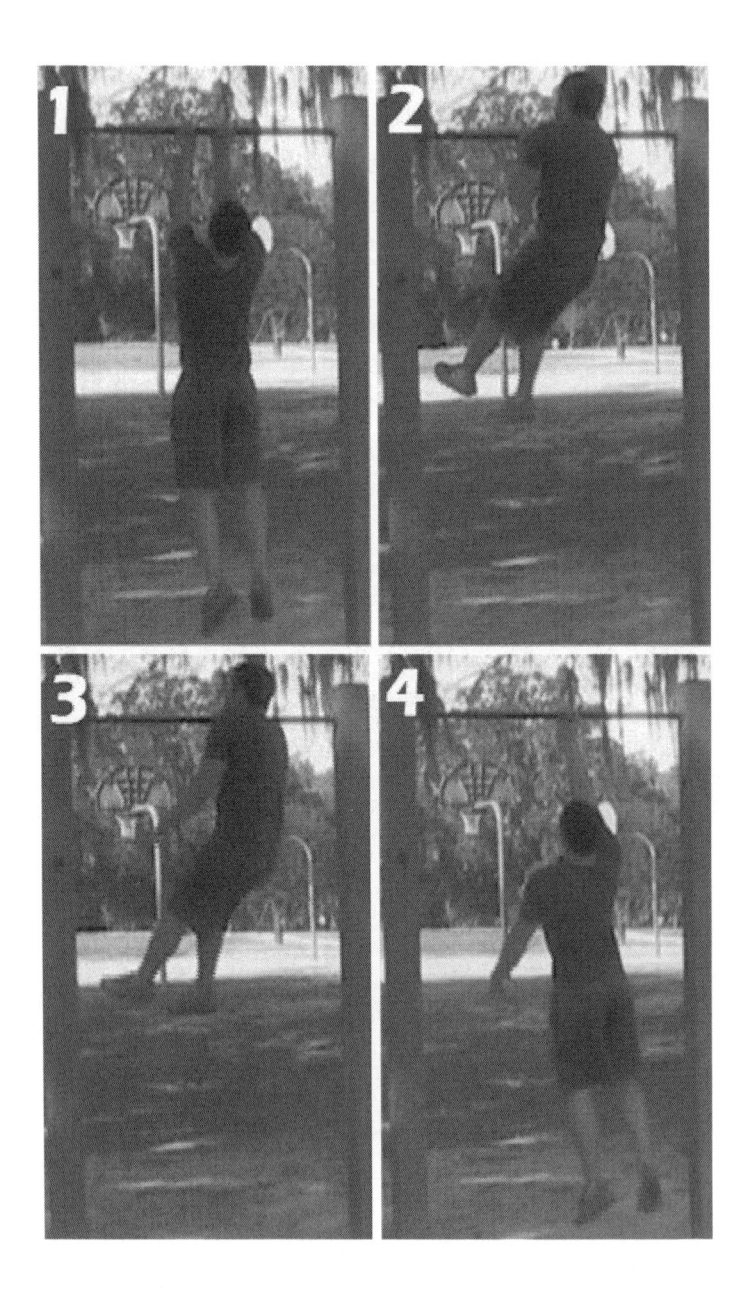

## One Arm Pull Up

In your first few workouts, I wouldn't recommend doing more than one rep per set on each arm, or doing more than two sets, just to see how your joints adjust. Again, this will be more of an issue for some people than for others depending on size, but you want to be careful.

If you feel like you're not in control, try not to let go of the bar on your way down and drop to the ground. Instead, bring your other arm up so that you have two hands on the bar, and then get down. While you're lowering yourself, your arm muscles are under a lot of strain—and so are your wrist, elbow, and shoulder joints.

If you release your grip on the way down, you go from being under a lot of strain to being under no strain in an instant, which can be painful and potentially dangerous. If you ever feel like you can't hold on with one hand, it's always better to return your other hand to the bar and get down from two hands instead of letting go with one.

If you are doing multiple reps, once you reach the full extension, put your secondary arm back on the bar, pull yourself back up to the top, and repeat the process. Don't get sloppy on your second and third (and so on) reps—always make sure that you are set and ready before you begin the negative.

As always, continue until you can no longer complete the exercise in a controlled and correct manner, and be sure to work both arms evenly.

One more thing I've learned—I used to feel like doing just one negative as slowly as I can was the best way to go about this. After trying both ways, I've since concluded that it's better to get in as many reps as you can as long as those reps are in good form. So, don't try to slow these reps down so you get more out of them—instead, aim to maximize the number of reps as long as you make sure to do them right and in good control.

## ONE ARM MIDWAY HANG

This is like the one arm version of the hang we talked about earlier in the book. Once you've gotten better at the one arm negatives, you can give these a shot.

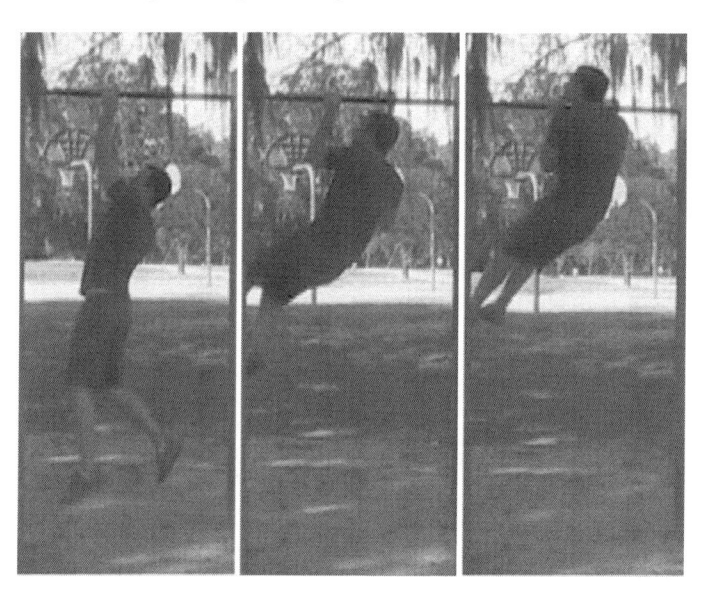

Basically, you're going to go through the same motions as you do in a one arm pull up negative, but you'll stop either at the top, middle, or bottom of the movement, and hold for as long as you can. Once you can't hold any longer, you lower yourself the rest of the way.

As an example, you might pull up on the bar with both hands, shift your weight to your left hand, let go of your right hand, and hold yourself at the top with just your left hand for as long as you can (could be just a second or two —that's fine).

Once you can't hold that any more, you lower yourself the rest of the way, then put your right hand on the bar, and then get off the bar and rest. After thirty seconds to a minute or so, pull back up, and do the same with your right hand instead of your left.

Then, rest, and repeat, except this time stop and hold the position when your upper arm is parallel to the ground, and then again lower yourself the rest of the way, then repeat with your other arm. Finally, repeat the whole thing a third time, this time holding the position (as with the two arm version) when your arm is almost fully extended but the muscles in your arm and back are still engaged.

## JUMPING ONE ARM PULL UP

This is basically one step removed from the one arm pull up, and it's the first exercise you'll do where you get your chin above the bar without using two arms.

Often, people who are trying to learn to do ordinary pull ups will train by jumping onto the bar and using that momentum to pull themselves all the way up. This kind of training can help them to achieve the regular pull up. Well, you're going to apply the same idea to the one arm pull up.

As we've been saying this whole time, the one arm pull up is much less stable than the ordinary pull up, and that's going to be important here. I would only recommend that you do this exercise on a bar that's low enough that you can grab the bar with one hand and still have your feet solidly on the ground. That way, when you jump, you're already holding onto the bar and you can begin pulling yourself up immediately.

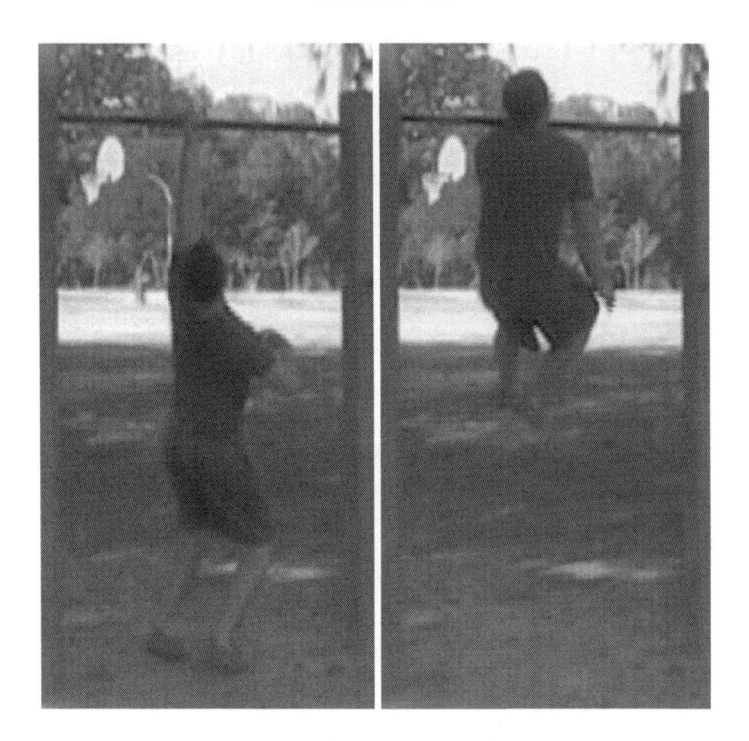

In other words, I don't want you to jump up, grab onto the bar in the air, and then try to establish control and pull yourself up. There are too many variables, and too much opportunity for you to get hurt. It's much better to work with a bar that will allow you to have a grip on the bar from the start.

You're going to grab onto the bar, give yourself a boost by bending your knees slightly and pushing off, and then immediately use that momentum to pull yourself straight above the bar. Then, lower yourself as you normally would when doing a one arm negative. As always, repeat until you can no longer properly execute the exercise, give yourself a minute or so, and then repeat with the other arm.

## One Arm Pull Up

Obviously, the harder you jump, the more help you're giving yourself. As you get stronger, jump less forcefully so that your arm will have to do more of the work. If you find yourself doing 6 or more of these, you need to give yourself less help, or start trying for the real thing.

# ONE ARM PULL UP

At this point, there's only one thing left to do. This will vary for everybody, but if you can do 6 consecutive one arm negatives or 6 consecutive jumping one arm pull ups, you're probably ready to give this a shot. Just get situated below the bar, grab onto it with one hand, take a breath, and squeeze and pull with every muscle involved from your hand, through your forearm and bicep, down through your back and even into your abs.

If you can get your chin solidly above the bar using only one hand, you are now in an elite club of strength athletes. Congratulations!

If you can't, don't worry. You've come a long way and you can definitely get there. Just go back to your routine for a couple more weeks, get stronger, and try again. Repeat until you get there.

One Arm Pull Up

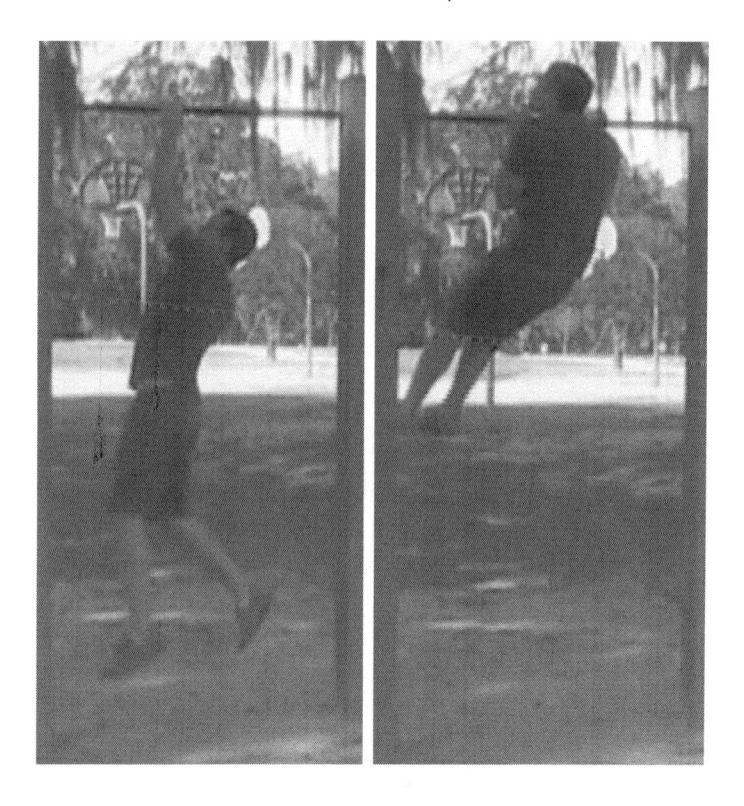

Oh, and don't kill yourself trying every day if you haven't gotten it yet. You'll just get more frustrated, and you almost definitely won't get there. If you can't do it, just get back to work and wait at least a couple of weeks to try again.

# REPS, SETS, AND SCHEDULES

One arm pull up workouts take quite a toll on your body, and—depending on your size, condition, schedule, and diet—I wouldn't recommend doing more than 2 workouts a week focused on acquiring this skill (if you're on the smaller side, and/or if you recover very quickly, you might think about doing three or more, but you need to use your own judgment on that).

At any rate, you don't ever want to do a one arm pull up workout if you're still feeling any muscle soreness or joint discomfort from your last one arm pull up workout, for the sake of avoiding injury.

For your workouts, you will follow a few basic guidelines:

1. Warm up thoroughly.

2. Do as much work as you can with the most difficult exercises you can do (the exercises are listed, more or less, in order of increasing difficulty).

3. Wait 2-3 minutes between exercises (experiment to see what period of rest allows you to do the most hard work in your workout).

4. Finish your workout with a set of pull ups and a set of chin ups to failure.

Important note: Stop your pull up work out if you experience joint pain. Try another workout in a few days once your joints and muscles recover.

The pattern you follow in your workouts will be different at different points in your progression. Let's take a look at how that pattern will evolve, starting with the beginning.

In the beginning, before you can do anything with one arm, your workouts will focus on the two arm exercises for your entire workout:

1. Warm up as described in the chapter on warming up.

2. Do the most difficult two arm pull up variation you can do for 1-3 sets.

3. When you can no longer do the previous exercise in good form, do the next-most difficult two arm pull up variation you can do for another 1-3 sets.

4. Do a set of midway hangs at each of the three major points in the range of motion.

5. Do a set of pullups and a set of chin ups to failure.

Once you can do a one arm pull up negative, one arm exercises will be the focus of your routine, although you will still do a lot of two arm exercises:

1. Warm up as described in the chapter on warming up.

2. Do the most difficult one arm pull up variation you can do for 1-3 sets.

3. When you can no longer do that exercise in a controlled manner, move to the next-most difficult exercise you can still do (one arm or two arm) for another 1-3 sets.

4. Do the most difficult two arm pull up variation you can for 1-3 sets.

5. Do a set of midway hangs at each of the three major points in the range of motion (one arm if possible, if not then two).

6. Do a set of pullups and a set of chin ups to failure. If you can do ten or more of either, you aren't working hard enough during the rest of your workout. You can also throw in one last pull up or chin up and try to do the slowest negative you can, for good measure, to finish the workout.

That might sound confusing, but you'll catch on quickly. It basically boils down to warming up, doing as much of the hard stuff as you can, doing some hangs for as long as you can hold them, and then doing some pull ups and chin ups to failure.

Once you start making some progress and getting the hang of things, you might want to add or change some exercises. Maybe instead of the hangs, you prefer to add in some slow negatives. That's fine. I would stick pretty close to what's recommended above in the beginning, but as long as you're following the basic structure and working as hard as you can (and doing as much one-arm focused exercise as you can), some substitutions can be fine.

With 2-3 minutes of rest between exercises, this workout can take a little while. It's a long time to spend doing pull ups, and you will be very sore afterward, especially as you progress and become able to do more work. Be sure to allow yourself to recover completely (muscles and joints) before doing your next one arm pull up workout.

As you get stronger, move on to harder and harder exercises and variations until you reach your goal.

To help you out once you're getting close, here's a sample of an "Almost There" workout you might find yourself doing:

1. Warm up.

2. 2 sets of eight pull ups, holding at the top and going down slowly on the last rep. Rest a couple of minutes in between.

3. 2 sets of jumping one arm pull ups, 5 reps each arm and then 4 reps each arm. 2 or 3 minutes rest between sets, and be sure to get the full negative in on the way down.

4. One arm midway hangs, one at each position for each arm for as long as you can. One minute or so in between each.

5. 1 set of biased pull ups, 1 set of biased chin ups on each arm. 5 reps each arm each set, two or three minutes between sets.

6. 1 set of pull ups to failure, 1 set of chin ups to failure (8 and 7 reps respectively). 3 minutes or so between sets.

7. One pull up or chin up with the slowest, steadiest negative you can manage on the way down.

The numbers will shift slightly one way or another depending on your size, but at that point, you should be exhausted. When you're getting close, these are the exercises you want to focus on—jumping one arm pull ups and biased pull ups, some hangs and some pull ups/chin ups to failure.

# ACTUALLY DOING
# A ONE ARM PULL UP

As you might expect, there's going to come a point when you're actually going to want to try to do a one arm pull up or chin up.

There's not a universal point at which you should start trying for a real one arm pull up, but as mentioned previously I would say that if you can do six one arm pull up (or chin up) negatives, or six jumping one arm pull ups or chin ups, then you could probably have a reasonable shot at the real thing.

As always, you want to make sure that you're thoroughly warmed up. You may even want to do an extra set or two of pull ups, including some slower pullups, to make sure you're totally warm—it might sound counter-intuitive, but it's better to be 'too' warmed up, to the point of almost being fatigued, than it is to be not warmed up enough, so don't be shy with the warm up exercises.

After you're warmed up, give yourself your 2-3 minute rest (whatever you've gotten used to at this point), and then get under the bar and give it a shot.

One thing to bear in mind, especially if you try it and fail, is that it might be a little difficult to get in a great workout after you've tried to do a one arm pull up or chin up. You should still finish the workout, but the point is not to get too tempted to try this every single time you go to the gym.

If all you keep doing is trying and failing to do a one arm pull up, it will become a distraction from the exercises that will actually help you make progress. If think you're close, but you try and fail, give yourself another couple weeks at least, or maybe even a month or so of good workouts before you try again.

# NUTRITION

This is an important topic to cover after discussing your scheduling, because nutrition is an absolutely vital part of your recovery which will impact whatever schedule you need to stick to.

Think about it. When your body is recovering, it's repairing itself. Imagine that you are trying to repair a house—you can't do it if you don't have the proper materials. The most talented repairman alive can't repair anything if he doesn't have the tools and materials for the job, and if he has low-quality tools and materials, he won't be effective either.

The same applies when we talk about repairing your body. For the quickest and most effective recovery (and the best health in general), you need to eat properly. This topic can fill a book, so we can't get in to too much detail here, but the most important thing that I would advise you to do is to eat real foods.

Food that is highly processed ends up in a state that is foreign to your body and totally unnatural. Your body has developed and evolved over the course of millennia, and it has adapted itself to the foods that were available over that time period.

Highly processed food products that have been invented in the past few decades are nothing like what your body has been built to process for thousands of years.

You aren't smarter than thousands of years of evolution, and neither is anybody working at those food and supplement companies. Your body is dazzlingly complex, and the muscle-building supplement some guy at your gym recommends to you could potentially be interfering with any number of other important things going on in your body.

Anything you buy that gets you 'results' quicker and bigger than your body can do on its own is going to have a trade-off that will catch up with you sooner or later—and when you're talking about a feat (like the one arm pull up) that requires strong joints as well as muscles, you don't want to develop your muscles out of proportion to your joints, because that can mean an injury.

The one arm pull up is not about looks, it is about human performance, and in my experience with trying to get my body to do its best, I always see the best results with natural foods. I don't use any powders or supplements, and I can't recommend that you do either.

I've written a book on my complete nutritional recommendations (*The Natural Diet*, available from Amazon.com and other retailers), but I'll summarize a few important ideas here:

1. Make fresh fruits and, to a lesser extent, fresh or cooked vegetables a large part of your diet.

2. Eat natural fats—a good rule of thumb is the fat should have an appetizing odor and flavor and should not require a factory for its production (butter, as well as peanut, olive, and coconut oil are good examples of natural fats you should eat).

3. Learn to read labels and avoid industrial food additives wherever possible.

4. Eat food in as close to its natural state as possible.

If you find yourself stalling out too much in your progress, it could be that you're not recovering properly and a poor diet may be to blame. Try to stick to these principles, and if you're interested in learning more, pick up a copy of *The Natural Diet*.

# CONCLUSION

The one arm pullup or chin up is an awesome target to pick. It's a challenge, and getting there will require you to work very hard, stay focused, and learn a lot about your body in the process—joints, limits, coordination, recovery, and so on.

Make sure you take advantage of all of the different pull up variations that you can do, both one arm and two arm. There will be times when you feel like one exercise is helping you make great progress, and suddenly you'll feel like you're just plateauing and getting nowhere. Experiment with the others, use good form, and you'll find another exercise to work into the routine that you love. Just keep working at it.

Even before you reach the goal of doing a one arm pull up, you will become much stronger in the process of training for one. You should see your grip strength and your ability to do regular pull ups increase considerably, and you will also develop many small muscles throughout your arm, back, and shoulder that are very difficult to hit without doing one arm training.

If I have one final piece of advice, it's just to stick with it. You're going to feel at times like you aren't getting anywhere, but as long as you're working as hard as you can without injuring yourself, you're getting closer. Remember that even if you can't do it yet, you're still getting much stronger.

This is a completely attainable goal for you. Just be patient, and be consistent, and you'll get there.

# BOOKS BY PATRICK BARRETT

*Natural Exercise: Basic Bodyweight Training and Calisthenics for Strength and Weight-Loss*

*The Natural Diet: Simple Nutritional Advice For Optimal Health In The Modern World*

*One Arm Pull Up: Bodyweight Training And Exercise Program For One Arm Pull Ups And Chin Ups*

# ABOUT THE AUTHOR

Patrick Barrett has been interested in exercise ever since he started to lift weights with his dad and older brothers as a kid. He participated in a half-dozen organized sports (most notably inline hockey and high school wrestling) until a neck injury during a wrestling match in his junior year prevented him from playing further in any contact sports.

After the injury, he developed an interest in pursuing strength and balance, particularly through bodyweight and self-taught gymnastic-type exercises.

Patrick has always loved both cooking and eating food. Unsatisfied with the confusing and often contradictory nutritional advice offered by mainstream sources, Patrick searched for another way to understand human nutrition that was logical, consistent, and effective. His books on food and nutrition reflect this 'cleaner,' more intuitive and useful understanding of food and how it impacts our health.

Patrick hopes that his books will save his audience time and aggravation by finally offering practical ways to achieve their nutrition and fitness goals.

Made in the USA
San Bernardino, CA
02 June 2014